MANAGING AND UNDERSTANDING MIGRAINE

A CLEAR PATH TO NAVIGATING AND CONTROLLING MIGRAINE

DANIEL ALEX

Contents

INTRODUCTION

In a world filled with diverse challenges and ever-evolving complexities, the pursuit of understanding and managing migraines takes center stage. Welcome to a journey that goes beyond the throbbing pain and visual disturbances, delving deep into the intricacies of migraines—a prevalent but often misunderstood neurological condition. This book, "Understanding and Managing Migraine: A Clear Path to Navigating and Controlling Migraine," aims to be your compass, guiding you through the labyrinth of information surrounding migraines and empowering you with the knowledge to seize control over this formidable foe.

Migraines, characterized by pulsating headaches and a range of sensory disturbances, affect millions worldwide, transcending age, gender, and cultural boundaries. Despite their prevalence, the true nature of migraines remains shrouded in mystery for many. This book embarks on a mission to unravel the intricacies of migraines, offering insights into the physiological and environmental factors that contribute to their onset. Through a comprehensive exploration of triggers and symptoms, we aim to equip you with the tools to decipher the unique language of your migraines.

As we venture into the realm of migraine management, this book adopts a holistic approach, recognizing the multifaceted nature of the condition. From traditional pharmaceutical interventions to integrative therapies and lifestyle adjustments, each chapter unveils a piece of the puzzle, providing you with a diverse toolkit to navigate the challenges posed by migraines. We delve into the significance of recognizing and mitigating triggers, empowering you to tailor a management plan that aligns with your individual needs.

Beyond the physical aspects, we acknowledge the profound impact migraines can have on one's emotional well-being and daily life. Strategies for maintaining mental resilience, fostering healthy relationships, and excelling in professional and social spheres are interwoven into the fabric of this exploration. Throughout this journey, you'll find not only practical advice but also a sense of community—a reminder that you are not alone in your quest for migraine understanding and control.

Embark with us on this odyssey, as we illuminate a clear path toward comprehending and managing migraines, paving the way for a life not dominated by pain but defined by resilience and control.

CHAPTER 1

OVERVIEW OF MIGRAINE

Migraine, a complex neurological condition, extends far beyond a mere headache—it is a dynamic interplay of genetic, environmental, and physiological factors that often remains elusive to those who grapple with its effects. This introductory exploration serves as a gateway into the intricate world of migraines, aiming to provide a comprehensive overview that transcends the common perception of throbbing head pain. From the diverse array of symptoms that accompany a migraine attack to the various triggers that can incite its onset, we embark on a journey of understanding the multifaceted nature of this prevalent yet enigmatic condition. Throughout this overview, we unravel the physiological intricacies of migraines, shedding light on the sensory disturbances, the role of neurotransmitters, and the distinct phases that characterize each episode. By establishing a foundation rooted in knowledge, we lay the groundwork for a deeper exploration into the nuanced aspects of migraine, empowering individuals to navigate their own unique experiences and fostering a greater understanding of this complex neurological phenomenon.

THE SIGNIFICANCE OF UNDERSTANDING MIGRAINE

Understanding migraine holds profound significance, as it transcends the realm of mere medical knowledge, reaching into the daily lives of individuals grappling with this neurological condition. The first layer of importance lies in dispelling the misconceptions that often surround migraines. While commonly associated with severe headaches, migraines encompass a spectrum of symptoms, including but not limited to visual disturbances, nausea, sensitivity to light and sound, and cognitive impairments. Recognizing this broad range of manifestations is crucial in fostering empathy and dismantling the stigma associated with migraines, as it establishes a more nuanced comprehension of the challenges faced by those affected.

Moreover, delving into the intricacies of migraine pathophysiology offers insights into the underlying mechanisms driving these attacks. The role of neurotransmitters, vascular changes, and genetic predispositions becomes apparent, contributing to a more holistic understanding of why migraines occur. This knowledge is not only empowering for individuals seeking to manage their condition but also forms the basis for targeted research and advancements in migraine treatment. As science unravels the molecular and genetic underpinnings of migraines, a deeper understanding paves the way for more effective therapies, potentially transforming the landscape of migraine management.

Beyond the physiological realm, comprehending migraines holds immense value in a socio-economic context. Migraine is a leading cause of disability worldwide, impacting productivity, work attendance, and overall quality of life. By understanding the socioeconomic implications, policymakers and employers can develop more compassionate and accommodating environments for those affected by migraines. This awareness becomes a catalyst for fostering inclusive practices that acknowledge the unique needs of individuals managing this condition, ultimately contributing to a more equitable and supportive society.

Furthermore, the significance of understanding migraine extends into the realm of mental health. The chronic nature of migraines can take a toll on one's emotional well-being, leading to anxiety, depression, and a sense of isolation. Knowledge about the psychological impact allows for the development of comprehensive care models that address both the physical and emotional aspects of migraines. In turn, this understanding aids healthcare professionals, support networks, and individuals themselves in implementing strategies to enhance mental resilience and improve overall quality of life.

In essence, grasping the complexities of migraine is not merely an intellectual pursuit but a transformative journey with far-reaching implications. From challenging societal perceptions to informing medical interventions, understanding migraine stands as a cornerstone in the pursuit of compassionate care, scientific progress, and an inclusive society that accommodates and supports those navigating the intricate landscape of migraines.

SETTING THE STAGE FOR EFFECTIVE MANAGEMENT

Setting the stage for effective migraine management is a pivotal initial step that involves creating a foundation for comprehensive care, tailored to the individual's unique experiences and needs. This process encompasses a multifaceted approach, addressing various aspects of the condition and the individual's lifestyle. Here are key components in establishing the groundwork for effective migraine management:

1. Accurate Diagnosis:
   - A precise and thorough diagnosis is fundamental for effective management. Consulting with healthcare professionals who specialize in neurology or headache medicine ensures a comprehensive evaluation of symptoms, potential triggers, and relevant medical history.

2. Education and Awareness:

- Knowledge is a powerful tool in managing migraines. Educating individuals about the nature of migraines, including common symptoms, triggers, and the potential impact on daily life, fosters awareness and empowerment. This understanding helps individuals make informed decisions about their care.

3. Personalized Treatment Plans:
- Recognizing the heterogeneity of migraines, healthcare providers should collaborate with patients to develop personalized treatment plans. This involves considering the frequency and severity of attacks, identifying triggers, and tailoring interventions to address individual needs. Treatment plans may include lifestyle modifications, medications, and alternative therapies.

4. Lifestyle Modifications:
- Lifestyle factors play a significant role in migraine management. Addressing aspects such as sleep patterns, dietary choices, stress management, and regular exercise can contribute to a more holistic and effective approach. Identifying and modifying specific triggers unique to the individual is crucial.

5. Medication Management:
- Medications are often a key component in managing migraines. Preventive medications may be prescribed to reduce the frequency and severity of attacks, while acute medications help alleviate symptoms during an episode. The choice of medications should be guided by the individual's medical history and the nature of their migraines.

6. Regular Monitoring and Adjustment:
- Migraines can evolve over time, and the effectiveness of treatments may change. Regular monitoring of symptoms, triggers, and treatment responses allows for adjustments to the management plan as needed. This ongoing collaboration between the individual and healthcare provider is essential for optimal care.

7. Psychological Support:

- Recognizing the emotional and psychological impact of migraines is integral to effective management. Incorporating psychological support, such as counseling or stress-reduction techniques, can enhance overall well-being and resilience in the face of migraine challenges.

8. Patient Empowerment:
   - Encouraging individuals to actively participate in their migraine management fosters a sense of control and empowerment. This involves open communication with healthcare providers, adherence to treatment plans, and the utilization of tools for self-monitoring and tracking.

In conclusion, setting the stage for effective migraine management is a collaborative and dynamic process that encompasses accurate diagnosis, education, personalized treatment plans, lifestyle modifications, medication management, regular monitoring, psychological support, and patient empowerment. By addressing these components comprehensively, individuals can lay the groundwork for a more proactive and successful approach to living with migraines.

CHAPTER 2

DECODING MIGRAINES

Decoding migraines requires unraveling the intricate language of a neurological phenomenon that extends beyond the realm of mere headaches. In this exploration, we embark on a journey into the complexities of migraines, seeking to decipher the unique patterns, triggers, and manifestations that characterize this often elusive condition. Beyond the pulsating pain, migraines reveal themselves as dynamic events with distinct phases, neurological intricacies, and a myriad of associated symptoms. By delving into the physiological and environmental factors at play, we endeavor to bring clarity to the enigma of migraines, empowering individuals with the knowledge to navigate their experiences and fostering a deeper understanding of the mechanisms underlying this prevalent and impactful neurological disorder.

ANATOMY OF A MIGRAINE ATTACK

The anatomy of a migraine attack involves a complex interplay of neurological and vascular processes, contributing to the characteristic symptoms experienced by individuals during an episode. While the exact mechanisms remain the subject of ongoing research, several key elements define the stages and physiological changes associated with migraines.

1. Prodrome Phase:
   - The prodrome phase serves as an early warning system, occurring hours to days before the onset of the actual headache. During this phase, individuals may experience subtle changes such as mood swings, increased sensitivity to light or sound, food cravings, or heightened irritability. These prodromal symptoms vary widely among

individuals and provide an opportunity for early recognition and intervention.

2. Aura Phase:
   - Not all individuals with migraines experience an aura, but for those who do, it typically precedes the headache. Auras are transient neurological symptoms that often manifest as visual disturbances, such as flashing lights, zigzag lines, or temporary vision loss. Other sensory disturbances, such as tingling or numbness, may also occur. The aura phase is thought to result from cortical spreading depression—a wave of neuronal hyperactivity followed by suppression—across the visual cortex.

3. Headache Phase:
   - The headache phase is the most recognizable and debilitating aspect of a migraine attack. It is characterized by a throbbing or pulsating pain, usually on one side of the head, although it can affect both sides. The intensity of the headache varies, and accompanying symptoms may include nausea, vomiting, sensitivity to light (photophobia), and sensitivity to sound (phonophobia). The headache phase can last from a few hours to several days.

4. Postdrome Phase:
   - Following the resolution of the headache, individuals may enter the postdrome phase, also known as the "migraine hangover." During this phase, individuals often feel fatigued, mentally foggy, and may experience lingering symptoms such as mild headache or irritability. The postdrome phase serves as a recovery period, and individuals gradually return to their baseline state.

The physiological basis of migraines involves the activation of the trigeminal nerve, release of neurotransmitters, and changes in blood flow within the brain. The trigeminal nerve releases neuropeptides, causing inflammation and dilation of blood vessels. This process is believed to contribute to the pain and other symptoms associated with migraines. Additionally, genetics, environmental factors, and individual triggers play roles in the susceptibility to migraine attacks.

Understanding the anatomy of a migraine attack goes beyond the surface-level perception of headaches, encompassing a cascade of intricate neurological events. By decoding these stages, researchers and healthcare professionals can develop targeted interventions and treatments to address the specific mechanisms underlying migraines, ultimately leading to more effective management strategies for individuals grappling with this complex neurological condition.

RECOGNISING DIFFERENT TYPES OF MIGRAINE

Recognizing different types of migraines is essential for accurate diagnosis and tailored treatment approaches. Migraines are not a one-size-fits-all condition; they manifest in various forms, each characterized by distinct symptoms and patterns. Understanding these different types enables healthcare professionals to provide more precise care, while individuals can better navigate their experiences. Here's an extensive exploration of some common types of migraines:

1. Migraine without Aura:
   - This is the most prevalent type of migraine. Individuals experience moderate to severe throbbing head pain, typically on one side, accompanied by symptoms such as nausea, vomiting, and sensitivity to light and sound. Unlike migraines with aura, there's no preceding visual or sensory disturbance in this type.

2. Migraine with Aura:
   - A significant subset of migraines involves an aura phase, where individuals experience temporary neurological symptoms before the headache begins. Visual disturbances, such as flashing lights or zigzag lines, are common, but auras can also manifest as sensory changes, language difficulties, or motor weakness. The aura phase usually lasts less than an hour.

3. Chronic Migraine:
   - Chronic migraines are characterized by experiencing headaches on 15 or more days per month, with at least eight of them fulfilling migraine criteria, for a minimum of three months. This type poses significant challenges due to its frequency, often leading to a heightened impact on daily life.

4. Menstrual Migraine:
   - Hormonal fluctuations, particularly around the menstrual cycle, can trigger migraines in some individuals. Menstrual migraines typically occur in the days leading up to, during, or after menstruation. Understanding the menstrual cycle's influence allows for targeted management strategies.

5. Vestibular Migraine:
   - Vestibular migraines involve dizziness and problems with balance, often without the severe headache. Individuals may experience vertigo, spatial disorientation, and unsteadiness. These symptoms can be debilitating and impact daily activities.

6. Ocular or Retinal Migraine:
   - Ocular migraines, also known as retinal migraines, involve temporary vision loss or visual disturbances in one eye. These episodes are usually short-lived and resolve on their own. However, they require prompt medical attention to rule out other potential causes.

7. Aura without Headache:
   - In some cases, individuals may experience an aura without the subsequent headache. This phenomenon is known as an aura without headache or a "silent migraine." The neurological symptoms occur, but the pain phase may be absent or minimal.

8. Status Migrainosus:
   - This represents an exceptionally prolonged and severe migraine attack, lasting for more than 72 hours. Status migrainosus can lead to

dehydration, and it often requires medical intervention to break the cycle of the migraine.

Recognizing these diverse types of migraines involves paying attention to the unique symptoms and patterns associated with each. Tracking the frequency, duration, and triggers of migraines can provide valuable information for healthcare professionals to make an accurate diagnosis and tailor effective management strategies. A collaborative approach between individuals and healthcare providers is crucial in decoding the specific nuances of each person's migraine experience.

CHAPTER 3

UNRAVELING TRIGGERS

Unraveling the intricate web of triggers that contribute to migraines is a crucial endeavor in the quest for effective management and prevention. Welcome to the exploration of "Unraveling Triggers," where we embark on a journey to dissect the diverse array of factors that can initiate and exacerbate migraine attacks. Triggers are the catalysts that set the stage for neurological disturbances, leading to the throbbing pain and associated symptoms characteristic of migraines. In this comprehensive investigation, we delve into the physiological, environmental, and lifestyle elements that intertwine to form an individual's trigger landscape. By decoding these triggers, we empower individuals to proactively navigate their daily lives, make informed choices, and construct personalized strategies aimed at minimizing the impact of migraines. Join us as we unravel the intricacies of triggers, shedding light on the pathways that, once understood, pave the way toward a clearer and more controlled journey through the realm of migraines.

IDENTIFYING PERSONAL TRIGGERS

Identifying personal triggers is a pivotal step in the journey to effectively manage and minimize the impact of migraines. Each individual's trigger landscape is unique, influenced by a myriad of factors ranging from genetics to lifestyle choices. This comprehensive exploration focuses on the process of recognizing and understanding personal triggers, empowering individuals to take proactive measures in their migraine management:

1. Keeping a Migraine Diary:
   - A fundamental tool in identifying personal triggers is maintaining a detailed migraine diary. Documenting the timing, intensity, and

duration of each migraine episode, along with associated activities, food intake, sleep patterns, and environmental conditions, provides a foundation for recognizing patterns over time.

2. Tracking Dietary Influences:
   - Certain foods and beverages are known to trigger migraines in susceptible individuals. Common culprits include caffeine, alcohol, chocolate, aged cheeses, and processed foods containing additives like monosodium glutamate (MSG). By systematically eliminating and reintroducing these items, individuals can identify specific dietary triggers.

3.Monitoring Sleep Patterns:
   - Disruptions in sleep patterns, whether due to insufficient sleep or irregular sleep schedules, can contribute to migraine attacks. Recognizing the correlation between sleep disturbances and migraines allows individuals to prioritize consistent sleep hygiene practices as part of their management strategy.

4. Stress and Emotional Triggers:
   - Emotional stress is a well-established trigger for migraines. Identifying specific stressors, such as work pressure, family issues, or relationship dynamics, enables individuals to develop coping mechanisms and implement stress reduction techniques like mindfulness, meditation, or therapy.

5. Environmental Factors:
   - Sensitivity to environmental stimuli varies among individuals. Bright lights, loud noises, strong odors, and changes in weather can act as triggers. By noting the surroundings during migraine episodes, individuals can pinpoint specific environmental factors and take preventive measures, such as using sunglasses or earplugs.

6. Hormonal Influences:
   - For some individuals, hormonal fluctuations, particularly in women, can trigger migraines. Tracking the timing of migraines in relation to

the menstrual cycle provides insights into hormonal influences. Hormonal therapies or lifestyle adjustments may be considered to address these triggers.

7. Physical Activity and Exertion:
  - Intense physical exertion or sudden, vigorous exercise can trigger migraines in certain individuals. Recognizing the role of physical activity as a trigger allows for the adoption of a more gradual and controlled approach to exercise, minimizing the risk of triggering migraines.

8. Weather Changes:
  - Barometric pressure changes, extreme temperatures, and humidity fluctuations are environmental factors that can influence migraines. Noting the weather conditions preceding migraine episodes helps individuals anticipate and manage their exposure to these triggers.

9. Caffeine Consumption:
  - While some individuals find relief from migraines through caffeine consumption, others may experience migraines triggered by caffeine withdrawal or excessive intake. Monitoring caffeine consumption patterns and experimenting with adjustments can unveil its role as a potential trigger.

10. Consultation with Healthcare Professionals:
  - Seeking guidance from healthcare professionals, such as neurologists or headache specialists, can provide valuable insights into identifying triggers. Medical professionals may recommend additional diagnostic tests, such as allergy assessments or hormonal evaluations, to uncover potential triggers.

In conclusion, identifying personal triggers requires a systematic and individualized approach. Through diligent self-observation, lifestyle adjustments, and collaboration with healthcare professionals, individuals can unravel the unique web of factors contributing to their migraines. Armed with this knowledge, they gain the power to make informed choices, implement preventive strategies, and pave the way toward more effective and personalized migraine management.

ENVIRONMENTAL FACTORS AND MIGRAINE

Environmental factors play a significant role in triggering and exacerbating migraine attacks. For individuals susceptible to migraines, understanding and managing these environmental influences are crucial components of an effective migraine management strategy. This comprehensive exploration delves into various environmental factors that can impact migraines:

1. Light Sensitivity (Photophobia):
   - Bright or flickering lights are common triggers for migraines. Fluorescent lighting, computer screens, and exposure to direct sunlight without adequate protection can provoke migraine episodes. Employing strategies such as using anti-glare screens, wearing sunglasses, or adjusting lighting conditions can help manage light sensitivity.

2. Noise Sensitivity (Phonophobia):
   - Loud or repetitive noises can trigger migraines in some individuals. Busy urban environments, construction sites, or even high-volume music may contribute to sensory overload. Wearing earplugs or noise-canceling headphones in noisy environments can mitigate this trigger.

3. Odor Sensitivity:
   - Strong odors, whether pleasant or unpleasant, can act as triggers. Perfumes, cleaning chemicals, smoke, and certain scents may provoke migraines. Identifying and avoiding specific odors, maintaining well-ventilated spaces, and using unscented products can help manage odor-related triggers.

4. Weather Changes:

- Fluctuations in weather conditions, such as changes in barometric pressure, extreme temperatures, or humidity, are recognized triggers for migraines. Sudden weather shifts, common during seasonal changes or storms, can be challenging to control but understanding their influence allows individuals to anticipate and prepare for potential migraine attacks.

5. Altitude Changes:
   - Changes in altitude, such as during air travel or mountainous terrain, can impact atmospheric pressure and trigger migraines. Staying hydrated and acclimatizing gradually to changes in altitude may help mitigate this environmental trigger.

6. Visual Stimuli:
   - Visual stimuli, such as rapidly moving patterns, intense visual stimuli (e.g., flashing lights), or prolonged screen time, can contribute to migraines. Individuals susceptible to migraines may benefit from minimizing exposure to such stimuli, taking breaks during screen use, and avoiding environments with intense visual displays.

7. Sleep Disruptions:
   - Environmental factors affecting sleep, such as noise, light, or an uncomfortable sleep environment, can influence migraines. Establishing a sleep-friendly environment, using blackout curtains, and maintaining a consistent sleep schedule contribute to better sleep quality and potentially reduce migraine occurrences.

8. Electromagnetic Exposure:
   - Some individuals report sensitivity to electromagnetic fields (EMFs) from electronic devices. While the scientific evidence on this topic is limited, individuals concerned about EMF exposure may choose to minimize screen time, keep electronic devices at a distance during sleep, or use devices that emit lower levels of electromagnetic radiation.

9. Allergens:

- Environmental allergens, such as pollen, dust, or pet dander, can trigger migraines in susceptible individuals. Identifying and minimizing exposure to specific allergens, using air purifiers, and maintaining a clean living environment may help manage this trigger.

10. Caffeine Intake:
    - While caffeine is often considered a potential trigger, it can also act as a remedy for some individuals. The source, amount, and timing of caffeine intake can influence its impact on migraines. Experimenting with caffeine consumption and observing its effects can provide insights into its role as a potential environmental trigger.

In conclusion, environmental factors exert a profound influence on migraines, and recognizing these triggers is instrumental in developing effective management strategies. By carefully observing and adapting to one's surroundings, individuals can gain better control over their environment, ultimately reducing the frequency and severity of migraine attacks. This proactive approach, combined with personalized lifestyle adjustments, empowers individuals to navigate the complexities of environmental triggers and enhance their overall quality of life.

CHAPTER 4

MEDICATION AND TREATMENT OPTIONS

Embarking on the labyrinth of migraine management involves a multifaceted approach, and at its core lies the realm of medication and treatment strategies. Welcome to an exploration that navigates the diverse landscape of options designed to alleviate the burden of migraines. From preventive measures aiming to reduce the frequency and intensity of attacks to acute treatments providing relief during an episode, this journey unfolds with the goal of empowering individuals to regain control over their lives. In this introductory exploration of medication and treatment, we delve into the pharmacological interventions, lifestyle adjustments, and holistic therapies that constitute the arsenal against migraines. Join us on a path that aims not only to mitigate the immediate pain but also to foster long-term strategies for a life less dominated by migraines and more characterized by resilience and well-being.

PHARMACEUTICAL APPROACHES

Pharmaceutical approaches to migraine management encompass a range of medications designed to either prevent the onset of migraines or alleviate symptoms during an attack. These medications target different aspects of the complex neurological processes underlying migraines. The extensive array of pharmaceutical options offers individuals and healthcare professionals the flexibility to tailor treatment plans based on the frequency, severity, and specific characteristics of the migraines.

1. Preventive Medications:
   - Preventive medications are prescribed to reduce the frequency and severity of migraine attacks. These include beta-blockers (e.g.,

propranolol), anticonvulsants (e.g., topiramate), tricyclic antidepressants (e.g., amitriptyline), and certain blood pressure medications. Botulinum toxin injections are also used for chronic migraine prevention.

2. Abortive or Acute Medications:
   - Abortive medications aim to stop a migraine attack once it has begun. Triptans, such as sumatriptan, are a common class of abortive medications that work by constricting blood vessels and blocking pain pathways in the brain. Other abortive options include nonsteroidal anti-inflammatory drugs (NSAIDs) like ibuprofen, and analgesics such as acetaminophen.

3. Combination Medications:
   - Some medications combine multiple active ingredients to address different aspects of migraine symptoms. For example, combination medications may include a pain reliever, a vasoconstrictor, and sometimes caffeine. These combinations can enhance the effectiveness of treatment for certain individuals.

4. CGRP Inhibitors:
   - Calcitonin Gene-Related Peptide (CGRP) inhibitors represent a relatively recent class of medications specifically developed for migraine prevention. These monoclonal antibodies target the CGRP pathway, which is implicated in migraine attacks. Aimovig, Emgality, and Ajovy are examples of CGRP inhibitors.

5. Ditans and Lasmiditan:
   - Ditans, such as lasmiditan, are serotonin receptor agonists designed for acute migraine treatment. Lasmiditan specifically targets serotonin receptors without causing blood vessel constriction, making it an option for individuals who cannot tolerate triptans or have cardiovascular concerns.

6. Antiemetics:
   - Antiemetic medications are prescribed to manage nausea and vomiting associated with migraines. Medications like metoclopramide

or prochlorperazine can provide relief from these gastrointestinal symptoms during an attack.

7. Corticosteroids:
- In certain cases, corticosteroids may be prescribed for short-term use to break a prolonged migraine attack or reduce inflammation associated with migraines. However, due to potential side effects, their use is generally limited to specific situations.

8. Rescue Medications:
- Rescue medications, such as medications containing butalbital, acetaminophen, and caffeine, are used on a limited basis to manage severe, infrequent migraines. However, their use is carefully monitored due to the risk of medication overuse headaches and dependency.

9. Hormonal Therapies:
- Hormonal therapies, including oral contraceptives or hormone replacement therapy, may be considered for individuals whose migraines are influenced by hormonal fluctuations. However, their use requires careful assessment of individual risk factors.

It is crucial for individuals to work closely with healthcare professionals to determine the most appropriate pharmaceutical approach for their specific situation. Tailoring treatment plans to individual needs, considering potential side effects, and monitoring the effectiveness of medications over time are essential components of successful pharmaceutical approaches to migraine management. Regular communication between patients and healthcare providers allows for adjustments and optimization of treatment strategies based on the dynamic nature of migraines and individual responses to medications.

INTEGRATIVE AND HOLISTIC APPROACHES

Integrative and holistic approaches to migraine management embrace a broader perspective, recognizing the interconnectedness of physical, mental, and emotional well-being. These strategies complement traditional pharmaceutical interventions, offering individuals a comprehensive toolkit to address various aspects of their health. From lifestyle modifications to alternative therapies, integrative and holistic approaches empower individuals to actively participate in their migraine management, fostering a sense of balance and resilience. Here's an in-depth exploration of key components within integrative and holistic migraine care:

1. Nutritional and Dietary Considerations:
   - Adopting a migraine-friendly diet involves identifying and avoiding potential trigger foods. Common dietary triggers include caffeine, alcohol, processed foods, and certain additives. On the flip side, incorporating nutrient-rich, anti-inflammatory foods, such as fruits, vegetables, and omega-3 fatty acids, may have a positive impact on migraine prevention.

2. Hydration and Fluid Balance:
   - Maintaining proper hydration is crucial for migraine management. Dehydration can trigger headaches, and individuals are encouraged to stay well-hydrated by drinking an adequate amount of water throughout the day. Monitoring and adjusting fluid intake based on individual needs and environmental conditions contribute to overall well-being.

3. Regular Exercise:

   - Engaging in regular physical activity has been shown to have a positive impact on migraine frequency and severity. Exercise promotes cardiovascular health, reduces stress, and releases endorphins, which can act as natural pain relievers. Tailoring exercise routines to individual preferences and capabilities is key to sustainability.

4. Sleep Hygiene Practices:

   - Establishing healthy sleep patterns is fundamental in migraine management. Consistent sleep schedules, creating a conducive sleep environment (e.g., dark room, comfortable bedding), and practicing relaxation techniques before bedtime contribute to improved sleep quality, reducing the risk of migraines.

5. Stress Reduction Techniques:

   - Stress is a well-established trigger for migraines. Integrative approaches emphasize stress reduction techniques such as mindfulness meditation, deep breathing exercises, yoga, and progressive muscle relaxation. These practices enhance resilience to stressors, promoting emotional well-being.

6. Acupuncture:

   - Acupuncture is an ancient Chinese therapy involving the insertion of thin needles into specific points on the body. Some individuals find relief from migraines through acupuncture, which is believed to balance the flow of energy (Qi) in the body. While research results are mixed, acupuncture is considered a low-risk intervention.

7. Biofeedback:
   - Biofeedback involves learning to control physiological functions, such as heart rate and muscle tension, to reduce migraine frequency and severity. Through monitoring and feedback, individuals gain awareness and control over involuntary bodily processes, enhancing their ability to manage migraines.

8. Herbal Remedies and Supplements:

- Certain herbs and supplements, such as butterbur, feverfew, magnesium, and riboflavin (vitamin B2), have been explored for their potential migraine-preventive properties. It's essential to consult with healthcare professionals before incorporating these into a treatment plan, as interactions and efficacy can vary.

9. Mind-Body Therapies:

- Mind-body therapies, including cognitive-behavioral therapy (CBT) and relaxation training, address the emotional and psychological aspects of migraines. These approaches help individuals identify and modify negative thought patterns, manage stress, and develop coping strategies.

10. Chiropractic Care:

- Chiropractic adjustments, particularly to the cervical spine, are sometimes explored as a complementary approach to migraine management. Research on the efficacy of chiropractic care for migraines is ongoing, and individual responses vary.

11. Aromatherapy:

- Aromatherapy involves the use of essential oils to promote relaxation and alleviate symptoms. Lavender, peppermint, and eucalyptus oils are commonly used for their potential calming and soothing effects. Individuals may experiment with aromatherapy to find scents that resonate positively with their well-being.

Integrative and holistic approaches to migraine management recognize the uniqueness of each individual's experience and encourage a proactive role in one's health. While these strategies may not replace pharmaceutical interventions, they provide valuable tools for enhancing overall well-being and resilience in the face of migraines. Collaboration with healthcare professionals ensures an integrative and holistic approach that aligns with individual needs and optimizes the potential benefits of these diverse strategies.

CHAPTER 5

LIFESTYLE ADJUSTMENTS

Navigating the realm of migraine management extends beyond medications and treatments, reaching into the sphere of lifestyle adjustments. In this journey, individuals discover the profound impact that everyday choices can wield in influencing the frequency and severity of migraines. Welcome to the exploration of lifestyle adjustments, where habits related to sleep, nutrition, stress, and daily routines become key players in the pursuit of a life with fewer migraines. Through a nuanced understanding of triggers and a commitment to fostering overall well-being, individuals embark on a proactive path, empowered to make informed choices that contribute to a more balanced and resilient lifestyle in the face of migraines.

DIETARY CHANGES FOR MIGRAINE MANAGEMENT

Dietary changes play a crucial role in migraine management, as certain foods and beverages can act as triggers for some individuals. Adopting a migraine-friendly diet involves identifying and modifying dietary patterns to reduce the risk of migraine attacks. While triggers can vary among individuals, common dietary culprits include:

1. Caffeine:

   - Caffeine can be a double-edged sword. While some find relief from migraines through caffeine consumption, sudden withdrawal can also trigger headaches. Moderation and consistency in caffeine intake, along with gradual reductions if needed, can help manage its impact.

2. Alcohol:

- Certain alcoholic beverages, particularly red wine, beer, and certain spirits, are known migraine triggers. Individuals prone to migraines may consider limiting or avoiding alcohol consumption to mitigate this potential trigger.

3. Tyramine-Containing Foods:
   - Tyramine, a naturally occurring compound, is found in aged and fermented foods. Cheese, cured meats, pickles, and fermented products can contain high levels of tyramine and act as triggers. Identifying and reducing the consumption of these foods is a common dietary adjustment.

4. Additives and Preservatives:
   - Some individuals are sensitive to additives and preservatives found in processed foods. Monosodium glutamate (MSG), nitrates, and nitrites are examples of additives that can trigger migraines. Choosing fresh, whole foods and reading labels carefully can help avoid these triggers.

5. Aspartame and Artificial Sweeteners:
   - Artificial sweeteners, such as aspartame, are potential triggers for some individuals. Opting for natural sweeteners or limiting the intake of products containing artificial sweeteners may be beneficial.

6. Chocolate:
   - Chocolate contains compounds like phenylethylamine and theobromine, which can influence blood flow and trigger migraines in susceptible individuals. While not universally problematic, some may choose to moderate their chocolate consumption.

7. Nitrates and Nitrites:
   - Found in cured meats, hot dogs, and processed foods, nitrates and nitrites are known triggers for some individuals. Selecting nitrate-free and minimally processed alternatives can be part of dietary adjustments for migraine management.

8. Citrus Fruits:

- Citrus fruits and juices contain histamine, which can be a trigger for some individuals. Monitoring the consumption of citrus fruits and exploring alternative sources of vitamin C may be considered.

9. Dairy Products:
 - A subset of individuals may be sensitive to dairy products. Experimenting with lactose-free or plant-based alternatives can help identify whether dairy is a potential trigger.

10. Gluten:
 - Some individuals with migraines may have gluten sensitivity. Exploring a gluten-free diet, with the guidance of healthcare professionals, can help identify whether gluten is a trigger for migraine attacks.

11. Dehydration:
 - Inadequate hydration can contribute to migraines. Ensuring sufficient water intake throughout the day, especially in warmer climates or during physical activity, is a fundamental dietary adjustment.

12. Migraine-Friendly Foods:
 - Incorporating nutrient-rich, anti-inflammatory foods can have a positive impact on migraine prevention. Fruits, vegetables, whole grains, lean proteins, and omega-3 fatty acids are examples of foods that contribute to overall well-being.

Individual responses to dietary changes can vary, and it's essential to approach these adjustments with mindfulness and patience. Keeping a detailed food diary, tracking migraine episodes, and seeking guidance from healthcare professionals, such as registered dietitians or neurologists, can provide valuable insights into the relationship between diet and migraines. Through a personalized and informed approach to dietary changes, individuals can proactively manage their migraines and contribute to an overall healthier lifestyle.

SLEEP HYGIENE AND IT'S IMPACT ON MIGRAINE

Sleep hygiene, encompassing a set of practices and habits that promote consistent and restful sleep, plays a pivotal role in migraine management. Disruptions in sleep patterns are not only a common trigger for migraines but can also exacerbate the severity and frequency of attacks. This comprehensive exploration delves into the impact of sleep hygiene on migraines and outlines key practices to foster better sleep quality:

1. Consistent Sleep Schedule:
   - Maintaining a regular sleep schedule involves going to bed and waking up at the same time every day, even on weekends. Consistency reinforces the body's internal clock, known as the circadian rhythm, promoting better sleep quality and reducing the risk of migraine triggers associated with irregular sleep patterns.

2. Creating a Sleep-Conducive Environment:
   - Designing a sleep-conducive environment involves keeping the bedroom cool, dark, and quiet. Blackout curtains, comfortable bedding, and minimizing noise can contribute to a relaxing atmosphere conducive to restful sleep, potentially reducing the likelihood of migraines.

3. Limiting Exposure to Screens Before Bed:
   - The blue light emitted by electronic devices like smartphones and computers can interfere with the production of the sleep-inducing hormone melatonin. Establishing a screen curfew, ideally one to two hours before bedtime, helps signal to the body that it's time to wind down, facilitating better sleep quality and potentially minimizing migraine triggers.

4. Mindful Eating Before Bed:

- Consuming heavy or spicy meals, caffeine, or alcohol close to bedtime can disrupt sleep and act as triggers for migraines. Adopting mindful eating practices, such as having a light evening snack if needed and avoiding stimulants, contributes to better digestion and sleep quality.

5. Regular Physical Activity:

- Engaging in regular physical activity promotes better sleep quality and can contribute to migraine management. However, exercising too close to bedtime may have a stimulating effect. Establishing a consistent exercise routine earlier in the day supports both overall well-being and improved sleep.

6. Relaxation Techniques:

- Incorporating relaxation techniques into the bedtime routine, such as deep breathing exercises, progressive muscle relaxation, or guided imagery, helps calm the mind and reduce stress. These practices contribute to better sleep quality and may mitigate migraine triggers associated with stress and tension.

7. Avoiding Excessive Napping:
- While short naps can be rejuvenating, excessive daytime napping can disrupt nighttime sleep. Limiting naps to 20–30 minutes and avoiding late-afternoon naps help maintain a healthy sleep-wake cycle, reducing the risk of migraines triggered by disrupted sleep patterns.

8. Managing Stress:

- Chronic stress is a significant migraine trigger, and its impact on sleep quality is profound. Implementing stress management techniques, such as mindfulness meditation, yoga, or journaling, can help manage stress levels and contribute to better sleep hygiene.

9. Limiting Caffeine in the Afternoon:

- Caffeine, a stimulant, can interfere with sleep when consumed too close to bedtime. Limiting caffeine intake in the afternoon and evening hours supports better sleep quality and reduces the risk of caffeine-related migraine triggers.

10. Addressing Sleep Disorders:

- Conditions like sleep apnea or insomnia can significantly impact sleep quality and contribute to migraines. Seeking evaluation and treatment for sleep disorders, when necessary, is crucial for comprehensive migraine management.

11. Establishing a Bedtime Routine:
- Creating a consistent bedtime routine signals to the body that it's time to wind down. Engaging in calming activities, such as reading a book, taking a warm bath, or practicing relaxation exercises, helps prepare the mind and body for restful sleep.

12. Seeking Professional Guidance:

- Individuals experiencing persistent sleep difficulties or migraines should seek guidance from healthcare professionals. Neurologists, sleep specialists, or other healthcare providers can conduct evaluations and provide personalized recommendations for managing sleep hygiene and migraines.

In conclusion, the intricate connection between sleep hygiene and migraines underscores the importance of fostering healthy sleep habits. By incorporating these practices into daily routines, individuals can create an environment conducive to restful sleep, potentially reducing the impact of sleep-related triggers on migraines. A holistic approach to migraine management, integrating sleep hygiene practices with other therapeutic strategies, empowers individuals to take control of their well-being and enhance their overall quality of life.

STRESS REDUCTION TECHNIQUES

Stress reduction techniques play a pivotal role in managing migraines, as stress is a well-established trigger for many individuals. The interplay between stress and migraines is complex, involving both physiological and psychological factors. Incorporating effective stress reduction techniques into daily life empowers individuals to mitigate the impact of stressors and potentially reduce the frequency and severity of migraine attacks. This comprehensive exploration delves into various stress reduction strategies:

1. Mindfulness Meditation:
   - Mindfulness meditation involves cultivating a heightened awareness of the present moment. By focusing on breath, sensations, or a specific point of focus, individuals can reduce stress and promote a sense of calm. Mindfulness-based stress reduction (MBSR) programs have shown efficacy in both stress reduction and migraine management.

2. Deep Breathing Exercises:
   - Controlled breathing exercises, such as diaphragmatic breathing or paced breathing, activate the body's relaxation response. Deep, slow breaths can help regulate the autonomic nervous system, reduce muscle tension, and alleviate stress. Practicing deep breathing regularly provides a portable and accessible tool for stress reduction.

3. Progressive Muscle Relaxation (PMR):
   - PMR involves systematically tensing and then relaxing different muscle groups. This technique helps individuals become more aware of and release physical tension. Regular practice can contribute to overall relaxation and reduce the muscle-related components of stress that may trigger migraines.

4. Yoga:

- Yoga combines physical postures, breath control, and meditation to enhance flexibility, strength, and mental well-being. Numerous studies suggest that yoga can be an effective stress reduction tool and may contribute to the prevention of migraines. Various styles of yoga, including gentle or restorative practices, cater to different needs and abilities.

5. Biofeedback:

- Biofeedback involves monitoring and gaining control over physiological functions, such as heart rate and muscle tension, through real-time feedback. By learning to consciously influence these functions, individuals can reduce stress levels. Biofeedback has demonstrated effectiveness in managing migraines by addressing stress-related triggers.

6. Cognitive-Behavioral Therapy (CBT):

- CBT is a therapeutic approach that focuses on identifying and modifying negative thought patterns and behaviors. It provides individuals with practical coping strategies for stress reduction. CBT has shown efficacy in reducing the frequency and severity of migraines by addressing stress and its impact on migraine triggers.

7. Guided Imagery and Visualization:
- Guided imagery involves using mental imagery to evoke a state of relaxation and positive emotions. Visualization techniques can transport individuals to calming scenes or scenarios. Regular practice can enhance relaxation responses and provide a mental escape from stressors.

8. Tai Chi:
- Tai Chi is an ancient Chinese martial art that combines gentle movements, meditation, and deep breathing. It has been associated with reduced stress levels and improvements in overall well-being.

The slow, flowing movements make it accessible for individuals of various fitness levels.

9. Aromatherapy:
   - Aromatherapy involves using essential oils to stimulate the olfactory system, influencing mood and relaxation. Scents like lavender, chamomile, and peppermint are commonly associated with stress reduction. Incorporating aromatherapy into daily routines can be a simple yet effective strategy.

10. Massage Therapy:
   - Massage therapy not only addresses physical tension but also promotes relaxation and reduces stress. Regular massages can contribute to overall well-being and potentially decrease the likelihood of migraines triggered by muscular tension.

11. Regular Exercise:
   - Engaging in regular physical activity, such as walking, jogging, or cycling, releases endorphins, the body's natural stress relievers. Exercise can also improve sleep quality, enhance mood, and reduce overall stress levels, contributing to migraine management.

12. Time Management and Planning:
   - Effective time management and planning can help individuals navigate daily challenges and reduce the perception of stress. Prioritizing tasks, setting realistic goals, and breaking larger tasks into manageable steps contribute to a sense of control and empowerment.

Incorporating a combination of these stress reduction techniques into daily life offers a comprehensive approach to managing stress and, consequently, reducing the impact of stress-related triggers on migraines. It's essential for individuals to explore and tailor these strategies based on their preferences, needs, and lifestyle. Collaborating with healthcare professionals, such as psychologists or therapists, can provide additional guidance and support in developing an individualized stress reduction plan.

CHAPTER 6

NAVIGATING DAILY CHALLENGES

Embarking on the journey of navigating daily challenges is an inherent part of the human experience, requiring a blend of resilience, adaptability, and proactive decision-making. In this dynamic process, individuals confront a spectrum of obstacles ranging from routine tasks to unforeseen complexities. Navigating daily challenges involves not only problem-solving but also fostering a mindset that embraces growth and learning in the face of adversity. This exploration invites individuals to cultivate a proactive approach, equipped with tools such as effective time management, stress reduction techniques, and a resilient mindset. As we delve into the intricate fabric of daily challenges, we discover opportunities for personal growth, self-discovery, and the development of strategies that empower us to navigate life's intricate tapestry with grace and determination.

WORK AND MIGRAINE : STRATEGIES FOR SUCCESS

Navigating the intersection of work and migraines demands a strategic and proactive approach to ensure success and well-being in a professional setting. Migraines can present unique challenges, impacting productivity, job satisfaction, and overall quality of life. However, with the right strategies and accommodations, individuals can thrive in their careers while effectively managing migraines. This comprehensive exploration delves into various aspects of work and migraine, offering practical strategies for success:

1. Open Communication with Employers:
   - Establishing open communication with employers is crucial. Informing supervisors about migraine challenges allows for

understanding and potential workplace accommodations. Discussing triggers, symptoms, and effective communication channels helps create a supportive work environment.

2. Flexible Work Arrangements:
   - Exploring flexible work arrangements, such as telecommuting or flexible hours, can provide individuals with more control over their work environment and schedule. This flexibility accommodates varying energy levels and allows for better migraine management.

3. Optimizing Workspace Ergonomics:

   - Creating an ergonomic workspace can reduce physical strain and contribute to overall well-being. Adjusting chair height, monitor placement, and lighting conditions can minimize factors that might exacerbate migraines and enhance comfort during work hours.

4. Mindful Time Management:

   - Implementing effective time management strategies can help individuals prioritize tasks and allocate energy wisely. Breaking tasks into manageable segments, utilizing to-do lists, and incorporating breaks contribute to a balanced workload that minimizes stress.

5. Utilizing Assistive Technology:

   - Assistive technologies, such as screen filters, voice recognition software, or ergonomic accessories, can enhance comfort and efficiency in the workplace. Customizing technology tools to individual preferences minimizes potential triggers and supports productivity.

6. Establishing a Support System:

   - Building a support system within the workplace involves educating colleagues about migraines and creating a network of understanding individuals. Colleagues can offer assistance during migraine episodes, contributing to a more empathetic and collaborative work environment.

7. Regular Breaks and Stretching:
   - Incorporating regular breaks and stretching exercises into the workday prevents physical strain and encourages blood circulation. These practices not only promote overall well-being but also reduce the risk of migraines triggered by prolonged periods of sitting or tension.

8. Creating a Dark or Quiet Space:

   - For those sensitive to light or noise, establishing a designated dark or quiet space in the workplace can serve as a retreat during migraine episodes. Employers may consider providing such spaces or allowing individuals to personalize their workstations for comfort.

9. Migraine Management Tools:

   - Leveraging migraine management tools, such as headache diaries or mobile applications, can help individuals track triggers, symptoms, and patterns. This data empowers individuals to make informed decisions about work-related adjustments and communicate effectively with healthcare professionals.

10. Implementing Stress Reduction Techniques:

   - Incorporating stress reduction techniques, such as mindfulness, deep breathing exercises, or quick relaxation routines, throughout the workday fosters resilience and reduces the impact of stress-related triggers on migraines.

11. Taking Advantage of Employee Assistance Programs (EAPs):

   - Many workplaces offer Employee Assistance Programs that provide resources for mental health and well-being. Utilizing these programs can connect individuals with counseling services, stress management resources, and additional support tailored to their needs.

12. Advocating for Workplace Policies:

   - Actively advocating for workplace policies that support individuals with migraines contributes to a more inclusive and accommodating work environment. Encouraging policies related to flexible scheduling, remote work options, and workspace adjustments benefits not only individuals with migraines but the overall workforce.

13. Seeking Professional Guidance:

   - Seeking guidance from healthcare professionals, such as neurologists or migraine specialists, ensures that individuals receive personalized advice and treatment plans tailored to their unique needs. Collaborating with healthcare professionals enhances the overall success of migraine management in the context of work.

Balancing work responsibilities and migraine management requires a proactive and collaborative approach that integrates individual needs with workplace accommodations. By implementing these strategies, individuals can foster a work environment conducive to success, well-being, and sustained career growth while effectively managing the impact of migraine.

SOCIAL LIFE AND MIGRAINE

Navigating a social life while managing migraines presents unique challenges, but with strategic approaches, individuals can foster meaningful connections, engage in social activities, and maintain overall well-being. Migraines can impact various aspects of social interactions, from planning activities to managing symptoms during social events. This comprehensive exploration delves into the intersection of social life and migraines, offering insights and practical strategies for a fulfilling and balanced social experience:

1. Open Communication with Friends and Family:

   - Establishing open communication with friends and family is key. Sharing information about migraines, triggers, and potential symptoms helps create understanding and empathy. Loved ones can offer support and adjust plans when needed, contributing to a more inclusive social environment.

2. Planning Social Activities Mindfully:

   - Mindful planning of social activities involves considering potential triggers and energy levels. Opting for activities with flexible timelines, manageable noise levels, and minimal stressors can enhance the overall social experience. Communicating preferences with friends ensures collaborative planning.

3. Building a Supportive Social Network:

   - Cultivating a supportive social network involves surrounding oneself with understanding individuals. Friends who are aware of migraine challenges can offer assistance during episodes and provide emotional support. Participating in group activities or support networks can foster connections with like-minded individuals.

4. Selecting Migraine-Friendly Venues:

   - Choosing social venues with considerations for potential migraine triggers contributes to a more comfortable experience. Opting for well-lit, well-ventilated spaces, or venues with quiet corners allows individuals to manage sensory sensitivities during social events.

5. Educating Friends About Migraines:

- Education is a powerful tool in fostering understanding. Providing friends with resources or information about migraines helps dispel misconceptions and promotes a supportive social environment. Knowledgeable friends are more likely to accommodate and empathize with migraine-related challenges.

6. implementing   Personal Boundaries:
   - Establishing and communicating personal boundaries is essential. Friends who are aware of an individual's need for occasional rest, quiet time, or specific accommodations can contribute to an environment that respects individual well-being and minimizes the impact of migraines.

7. Having a Migraine Toolkit:

   - Preparing a migraine toolkit for social outings includes items such as pain relievers, sunglasses, earplugs, and water. Being equipped with these essentials allows individuals to manage symptoms proactively, providing a sense of control during social activities.

8. Utilizing Technology for Social Connection:

   - Leveraging technology allows individuals to maintain social connections even during times when in-person interactions might be challenging. Video calls, messaging apps, and virtual gatherings offer alternatives for staying connected without the potential triggers associated with physical gatherings.

9. Prioritizing Self-Care After Social Activities:

   - Recognizing the importance of self-care after social activities is crucial. Taking time to rest, practice relaxation techniques, or engage in activities that bring comfort helps manage potential post-social fatigue or migraine triggers.

10. Exploring Migraine-Friendly Hobbies:

   - Pursuing hobbies that align with individual preferences and migraine management goals can contribute to a fulfilling social life. Whether it's joining a book club, engaging in creative pursuits, or participating in low-intensity physical activities, finding enjoyable and migraine-friendly hobbies enhances social well-being.

11. Advocating for Personal Needs:

   - Advocating for personal needs within social circles involves expressing preferences and communicating openly about migraine-related considerations. Friends who understand and respect individual needs contribute to a social environment that accommodates rather than exacerbates migraine challenges.

12. Engaging in Social Activities Gradually:

   - Gradual engagement in social activities allows individuals to build tolerance and resilience. Starting with shorter outings or smaller gatherings and gradually increasing social interactions can help manage energy levels and potential triggers.

13. Seeking Professional Support:
   - Seeking support from healthcare professionals, such as therapists or support groups, can provide guidance on managing the emotional and psychological aspects of living with migraines. Professional support contributes to overall well-being and resilience in social interactions.

Balancing a social l life while managing migraines involves intentional planning, effective communication, and a commitment to self-care. By implementing these strategies, individuals can foster meaningful connections, cultivate understanding within social circles, and enjoy a fulfilling social life while effectively managing the impact of migraines.

CHAPTER 7

EMPOWERING CONTROL

Empowering control is a journey of self-discovery and intentional action, where individuals take charge of their lives, decisions, and well-being. It involves cultivating a mindset that embraces personal agency, resilience, and the capacity to navigate challenges with a sense of purpose. Empowering control is not about eliminating uncertainties but rather about developing the tools and strategies to respond effectively to them. It encompasses the proactive pursuit of goals, the ability to make informed choices, and the resilience to adapt to changing circumstances. As individuals embark on the path of empowering control, they discover the transformative strength that arises from self-awareness, intentional decision-making, and the recognition that they possess the ability to shape their own narratives.

DEVELOPING A PERSONALIZED MIGRAINE MANAGEMENT PLAN

Developing a personalized migraine management plan is a vital and empowering process that allows individuals to take control of their well-being, identify triggers, and implement effective strategies for prevention and relief. This comprehensive exploration delves into the key components of creating a personalized migraine management plan:

1. Diagnosis and Assessment:

   - The foundation of a personalized migraine management plan begins with a thorough diagnosis and assessment. Consulting with a healthcare professional, typically a neurologist or headache specialist, helps confirm the migraine diagnosis, understand the individual's unique symptoms, and assess the frequency and severity of attacks.

2. Trigger Identification:

   - Identifying triggers is a critical step in tailoring a management plan. Keeping a detailed migraine diary that includes information on food and drink consumption, sleep patterns, stress levels, environmental factors, and other potential triggers helps individuals recognize patterns and pinpoint specific triggers that contribute to migraine attacks.

3. Lifestyle Modifications:

   - Based on trigger identification, lifestyle modifications become an integral part of the management plan. This includes adjustments to sleep patterns, dietary choices, stress management techniques, and physical activity. Tailoring these modifications to individual preferences and needs ensures a sustainable and personalized approach to migraine prevention.

4. Medication Management:

   - For many individuals, medication is a crucial component of migraine management. Working closely with healthcare professionals helps determine the most suitable medications for prevention and relief. This may include acute medications to address symptoms during an attack and preventive medications to reduce the frequency and severity of migraines.

5. Establishing a Routine:

   - Creating a daily routine provides a sense of stability and predictability, contributing to overall migraine management. This includes consistent sleep patterns, regular meals, hydration, and the incorporation of stress reduction techniques into daily life. Routine helps minimize potential triggers and enhances the effectiveness of preventive measures.

6.Coping Strategies:

- Developing effective coping strategies is essential for dealing with the impact of migraines on mental and emotional well-being. Mindfulness meditation, relaxation exercises, and cognitive-behavioral techniques can be incorporated into the management plan to enhance resilience and reduce the emotional toll of migraines.

7. Environmental Considerations:

- Evaluating and addressing environmental factors that may contribute to migraines is crucial. This includes minimizing exposure to strong odors, managing lighting conditions, and creating a comfortable workspace. Environmental considerations contribute to a personalized approach that takes into account an individual's unique sensitivities.

8. Regular Monitoring and Adjustments:

- A dynamic migraine management plan requires regular monitoring and adjustments. Periodically reviewing the effectiveness of lifestyle modifications, medications, and coping strategies allows individuals to make informed adjustments based on changes in triggers, symptoms, or overall well-being.

9. Education and Awareness:

- Educating oneself about migraines, their triggers, and available treatments fosters empowerment. Understanding the nature of migraines and staying informed about new developments in migraine research contributes to a proactive and informed approach to management.

10. Social Support and Communication:

- Incorporating social support into the management plan involves communicating with friends, family, and colleagues about migraine challenges. Sharing information about individual needs, triggers, and potential accommodations helps create a supportive network that understands and respects the individual's journey.

11. Emergency Plan:
- Developing an emergency plan ensures preparedness for severe migraine attacks. This may include communication strategies with employers, a plan for accessing medical assistance, and having necessary medications and comfort measures readily available.

12. Professional Guidance:
- Seeking ongoing guidance from healthcare professionals, including neurologists, headache specialists, and mental health professionals, is essential. Regular check-ins allow for the assessment of progress, adjustments to treatment plans, and addressing any emerging challenges.

In conclusion, developing a personalized migraine management plan is a holistic and ongoing process that embraces individuality and adaptability. By integrating medical, lifestyle, and psychological components, individuals can craft a comprehensive approach that empowers them to navigate the complexities of migraines with resilience, control, and an improved quality of life.

TRACKING AND ANALYZING MIGRAINE PATTERNS

Tracking and analyzing migraine patterns is a powerful tool that empowers individuals to gain insights into the triggers, symptoms, and trends associated with their migraines. This meticulous process involves the systematic recording of various factors, allowing for a comprehensive understanding of the unique characteristics of each migraine episode. The information gathered through tracking becomes instrumental in tailoring effective management strategies. This exploration delves into the importance of tracking and provides guidance on how to systematically analyze migraine patterns:

1. Migraine Diary Creation:
   - The foundation of tracking migraine patterns is the creation of a detailed migraine diary. This diary should include information such as the date and time of each migraine episode, the duration and intensity of the headache, associated symptoms (such as nausea or aura), and any identifiable triggers. Additionally, record details about sleep patterns, dietary choices, stress levels, and medication use.

2. Identifying Triggers:
   - Analyzing the migraine diary over time allows individuals to identify patterns and potential triggers. Triggers can vary widely among individuals and may include specific foods, hormonal changes, environmental factors, stressors, or sleep disturbances. By correlating migraine episodes with daily activities, individuals can pinpoint common denominators and gain insights into their unique triggers.

3. Recognizing Prodrome and Aura:
   - Tracking migraine patterns enables individuals to recognize prodromal symptoms and auras that precede the onset of a migraine. Prodromal symptoms may include subtle changes in mood, energy levels, or cognition, while auras manifest as sensory disturbances. Recognizing these early signs provides a window of opportunity for proactive management and preventive measures.

4. Monitoring Medication Efficacy:
   - For those using migraine medications, tracking their effectiveness is crucial. Record the type and dosage of medications taken during each episode, along with their impact on symptom relief. This information helps healthcare professionals assess the effectiveness of current medications and explore adjustments if needed.

5. Assessing Frequency and Duration:

- Analyzing the frequency and duration of migraine episodes provides a quantitative perspective on migraine patterns. Individuals can identify trends, such as variations in occurrence during specific times of the month or seasonal changes. This information aids in setting realistic expectations and adjusting preventive measures accordingly.

6. Sleep and Lifestyle Analysis:
   - Examining sleep patterns and lifestyle factors contributes to a holistic understanding of migraine patterns. Analyze data related to sleep duration, sleep quality, and daily routines to identify potential correlations with migraine episodes. Lifestyle adjustments, such as regular sleep schedules and stress management, can then be refined based on this analysis.

7. Weather and Environmental Factors:
   - Some individuals are sensitive to weather changes or specific environmental factors. Recording weather conditions and potential triggers in the environment, such as strong odors or bright lights, aids in identifying external influences on migraines. Adjustments to daily routines or activities can be made based on these insights.

8. Emotional and Stress Analysis:
   - Emotional well-being and stress levels significantly impact migraines. Analyze the migraine diary for patterns related to stressors, emotional fluctuations, and lifestyle stress. Recognizing these connections facilitates the implementation of effective stress management techniques as part of a comprehensive migraine management plan.

9. Trend Analysis over Time:
   - Regularly reviewing the migraine diary allows for trend analysis over time. Individuals can identify improvements or exacerbations in migraine patterns and assess the effectiveness of implemented interventions. This ongoing analysis informs adjustments to the management plan, ensuring its relevance to the current state of migraine patterns.

10. Seeking Professional Guidance:
  - While tracking and analyzing migraine patterns provide valuable self-insights, consulting with healthcare professionals is essential. Neurologists or headache specialists can offer guidance on interpreting patterns, adjusting medications, and implementing personalized interventions based on the collected data.

11. Utilizing Migraine Tracking Apps:
  - Migraine tracking apps can streamline the process by providing user-friendly platforms for recording and analyzing migraine patterns. These apps often include features for tracking triggers, symptoms, medication usage, and other relevant data, making it easier for individuals to maintain a comprehensive diary.

In conclusion, tracking and analyzing migraine patterns serve as indispensable tools in the proactive management of migraines. By systematically collecting and reviewing data, individuals gain a deeper understanding of their unique migraine characteristics, enabling them to make informed decisions, refine their management strategies, and work collaboratively with healthcare professionals for optimal migraine care.

SETTING REALISTIC GOALS FOR CONTROL

Setting realistic goals for migraine control is a fundamental aspect of proactive management that empowers individuals to navigate the complexities of migraine management effectively. Realistic goals provide a framework for progress, foster a sense of achievement, and contribute to an overall strategy that aligns with an individual's unique needs and circumstances. This comprehensive exploration delves into the importance of setting realistic goals for migraine control and offers guidance on establishing and achieving them:

1. Understanding Individual Triggers:
  - The first step in setting realistic goals for migraine control involves a deep understanding of individual triggers. Identifying and

acknowledging specific triggers, whether they are related to lifestyle, environment, or other factors, allows individuals to set goals that directly address the root causes of their migraines.

2. Collaborating with Healthcare Professionals:

   - Collaborating with healthcare professionals, such as neurologists or headache specialists, is crucial in defining realistic goals. Professionals can provide insights into the individual's medical history, prescribe appropriate medications, and offer guidance on lifestyle adjustments that align with specific migraine patterns.

3. Gradual Lifestyle Adjustments:

   - Setting realistic goals often involves gradual lifestyle adjustments. Whether it's implementing changes in sleep patterns, modifying dietary habits, or incorporating stress reduction techniques, taking gradual steps ensures that adjustments are sustainable and manageable.

4. Defining Short-Term and Long-Term Objectives:

   - Establishing both short-term and long-term objectives is essential. Short-term goals focus on immediate actions and changes, providing a sense of accomplishment and motivation. Long-term goals encompass broader outcomes and emphasize the sustained management of migraines over time.

5. Prioritizing Stress Reduction:

   - Stress is a common trigger for migraines, and prioritizing stress reduction can be a central goal. Realistic stress reduction goals may involve incorporating mindfulness practices, setting boundaries, and identifying effective coping strategies to manage stressors proactively.

6. Consistent Medication Management:

- For individuals using medications for migraine management, setting realistic goals involves consistent and appropriate medication management. This includes adhering to prescribed dosages, communicating effectively with healthcare professionals about medication effectiveness, and addressing any concerns or side effects promptly.

7. Monitoring and Adjusting Goals:

- Regular monitoring of progress allows for goal adjustments based on individual responses and evolving circumstances. Analyzing migraine patterns, lifestyle changes, and the effectiveness of interventions helps individuals refine their goals to ensure they remain realistic and relevant.

8. Embracing Flexibility:

- Flexibility is key in setting realistic goals, considering the unpredictable nature of migraines. Embracing a flexible mindset allows individuals to adapt their goals based on fluctuations in symptoms, unexpected triggers, or changes in personal circumstances.

9. Establishing a Sleep Routine:

- Sleep patterns significantly impact migraines, and establishing a consistent sleep routine can be a realistic and impactful goal. Prioritizing sufficient and quality sleep, along with creating a conducive sleep environment, contributes to overall well-being and migraine control.

10. Incorporating Regular Physical Activity:

- Setting realistic goals for physical activity involves incorporating regular, moderate exercise into the routine. This might include activities such as walking, yoga, or swimming, tailored to individual preferences and abilities. Physical activity contributes to overall health and can positively influence migraine management.

11. Building a Support Network:

   - Establishing a support network is a realistic goal that involves communicating with friends, family, and colleagues about migraine challenges. Building understanding and support within one's social circle can enhance overall well-being and contribute to effective migraine management.

12. Seeking Professional Guidance:

   - Seeking professional guidance is an essential aspect of setting realistic goals. Healthcare professionals can provide personalized advice, monitor progress, and collaborate on adjustments to the management plan based on the individual's unique responses and needs.

13. Celebrating Achievements:

   - Celebrating achievements, no matter how small, is crucial for maintaining motivation and reinforcing positive behaviors. Recognizing and acknowledging progress towards goals fosters a sense of accomplishment and encourages continued efforts in migraine control.

CHAPTER 8

EMOTIONAL WELLBEING

Emotional well-being is the cornerstone of a fulfilling and balanced life, encompassing the overall health and resilience of an individual's emotional state. It involves the ability to understand, express, and manage emotions effectively, fostering a positive and harmonious relationship with oneself and others. Emotional well-being goes beyond the absence of negative emotions; it embraces the cultivation of positive emotions, coping mechanisms, and a sense of purpose. Nurturing emotional well-being is a holistic endeavor that intertwines mental, social, and physical aspects of health, contributing to a resilient and adaptive mindset in the face of life's challenges. As individuals prioritize their emotional well-being, they embark on a journey towards self-discovery, self-compassion, and the pursuit of a more enriched and meaningful life.

ADDRESSING EMOTIONAL IMPACT

Addressing the emotional impact of various life challenges, including health conditions like migraines, is a crucial aspect of overall well-being. Emotional well-being is intertwined with mental health, and acknowledging, understanding, and managing emotions can significantly contribute to resilience and adaptive coping mechanisms. This comprehensive exploration delves into strategies for addressing the emotional impact of migraines and other challenges:

1. Acknowledging Emotions:

   - The first step in addressing the emotional impact of migraines is acknowledging and validating emotions. Whether it's frustration, anxiety, sadness, or any other feeling, recognizing and accepting these emotions as valid responses to the challenges of living with migraines is essential.

2. Open Communication:

- Engaging in open communication with oneself and others is a powerful tool in addressing emotional impact. Sharing feelings, concerns, and experiences with trusted friends, family, or healthcare professionals fosters a supportive environment and helps individuals feel understood.

3. Building Emotional Awareness:

- Building emotional awareness involves developing a deep understanding of one's emotional landscape. This includes recognizing triggers, identifying patterns of emotional responses, and gaining insight into how emotions may influence migraines. Increased awareness empowers individuals to make informed decisions about managing emotional well-being.

4. Seeking Professional Support:

- Professional support from mental health professionals, such as psychologists or counselors, can provide valuable guidance in addressing the emotional impact of migraines. Therapy offers a safe space to explore emotions, develop coping strategies, and navigate the psychological aspects of living with a chronic health condition.

5. Mindfulness and Relaxation Techniques:

- Mindfulness practices, including meditation and relaxation techniques, contribute to emotional well-being by promoting a present-moment awareness. These practices can help individuals manage stress, reduce anxiety, and cultivate a calm mindset, which may positively impact the emotional aspects of migraines.

6. Journaling and Reflection:

- Journaling serves as a therapeutic outlet for expressing emotions and reflecting on experiences. Writing about the emotional impact of migraines allows individuals to gain insights into their thoughts and feelings, facilitating a process of self-discovery and emotional processing.

7. Establishing Healthy Boundaries:

- Establishing and maintaining healthy boundaries is crucial for emotional well-being. This involves recognizing personal limits, communicating needs effectively, and advocating for oneself. Setting boundaries with work, social activities, and even healthcare interactions contributes to a balanced and sustainable emotional state.

8. Empowering Control:

- Empowering control over one's life and health journey is an effective strategy for addressing emotional impact. Setting realistic goals, taking proactive steps in migraine management, and making informed decisions contribute to a sense of agency and empowerment.

9. Building a Support System:

- Building a robust support system involves cultivating connections with understanding friends, family, or support groups. Having a network that acknowledges the emotional challenges of migraines provides a source of comfort, encouragement, and shared experiences.

10. Embracing Self-Compassion:

- Practicing self-compassion involves treating oneself with kindness and understanding, especially during challenging times. Acknowledging that living with migraines can be emotionally taxing and embracing self-compassion allows individuals to navigate their experiences with greater resilience.

11. Engaging in Enjoyable Activities:

- Engaging in activities that bring joy and fulfillment is a proactive way to address emotional impact. Whether it's pursuing hobbies, spending time with loved ones, or enjoying moments of relaxation, incorporating positive experiences contributes to emotional well-being.

12. Cognitive-Behavioral Techniques:

- Cognitive-behavioral techniques, guided by professionals, can help individuals identify and reframe negative thought patterns that may contribute to emotional distress. These techniques empower individuals to develop healthier perspectives and coping strategies.

13. Recognizing the Grief Process:

- Living with migraines can involve a grieving process for the life one envisioned. Recognizing and allowing oneself to move through the stages of grief—denial, anger, bargaining, depression, and acceptance—can be a transformative aspect of addressing the emotional impact.

14. Education and Empowerment:

- Educating oneself about migraines, triggers, and available treatments empowers individuals to make informed decisions. Knowledge acts as a tool for understanding the condition and its emotional aspects, contributing to a sense of control and mastery.

In conclusion, addressing the emotional impact of migraines involves a multifaceted approach that integrates self-awareness, communication, support, and proactive strategies. By adopting these strategies, individuals can cultivate emotional resilience, navigate the challenges of living with migraines, and enhance their overall well-being.

BUILDING RESILIENCE IN THE FACE OF MIGRAINE

Building resilience in the face of migraines is a transformative process that empowers individuals to navigate challenges, adapt to adversity, and maintain well-being despite the impact of chronic headaches. Resilience is not about eliminating the presence of migraines but rather developing the capacity to respond effectively, bounce back from setbacks, and cultivate a positive mindset. This comprehensive exploration delves into strategies for building resilience in the face of migraines:

1. Mindfulness and Acceptance:

   - Embracing mindfulness and acceptance is foundational to building resilience. Mindfulness practices, such as meditation and deep-breathing exercises, enable individuals to cultivate present-moment awareness and accept their experiences without judgment. This approach fosters a resilient mindset by reducing the emotional resistance to migraines.

2. Cognitive Restructuring:

   - Cognitive restructuring involves identifying and challenging negative thought patterns related to migraines. By reframing perceptions and cultivating a more positive outlook, individuals can build resilience in the face of chronic pain. This technique helps shift the focus from the limitations imposed by migraines to one's ability to cope and adapt.

3. Establishing a Support System:

   - Building a robust support system is integral to resilience. Connecting with friends, family, or support groups provides a source of understanding, empathy, and encouragement. Sharing experiences with individuals who comprehend the challenges of migraines fosters a sense of community and bolsters emotional resilience.

4. Goal Setting and Achieving:

   - Setting and achieving realistic goals contributes to a sense of accomplishment and resilience. Establishing both short-term and long-term goals related to migraine management, self-care, or personal growth allows individuals to focus on positive outcomes and reinforces their ability to navigate challenges effectively.

5. Adaptive Coping Strategies:

   - Developing adaptive coping strategies is essential for resilience. This involves identifying and implementing healthy ways to cope with stress, pain, and emotional challenges. Techniques such as relaxation exercises, creative outlets, or engaging in enjoyable activities serve as proactive tools in building resilience.

6. Creating a Positive Lifestyle:

   - Cultivating a positive lifestyle encompasses making choices that contribute to overall well-being. This includes maintaining a balanced diet, staying hydrated, prioritizing regular sleep, and incorporating physical activity into daily routines. A positive lifestyle serves as a foundation for physical and emotional resilience.

7. Learning from Challenges:

- Embracing a mindset of continuous learning from challenges enhances resilience. Each migraine episode can provide valuable insights into triggers, coping mechanisms, and personal strengths. Reflecting on these experiences fosters a growth-oriented perspective that contributes to increased resilience over time.

8. Embracing Flexibility:

   - Flexibility is a key component of resilience. Being adaptable in the face of unpredictable migraines involves adjusting plans, expectations, and strategies as needed. Embracing flexibility allows individuals to navigate the ebb and flow of migraine patterns with greater ease.

9. Seeking Professional Guidance:

   - Seeking guidance from healthcare professionals, such as neurologists or therapists, plays a crucial role in building resilience. Professionals can offer personalized strategies, coping techniques, and emotional support that contribute to an individual's ability to endure and bounce back from the challenges of living with migraines.

10. Developing a Sense of Purpose:
   - Cultivating a sense of purpose provides individuals with a motivational anchor that transcends the difficulties of migraines. Identifying personal values, passions, and meaningful pursuits creates a foundation for resilience and empowers individuals to persevere through challenging moments.

11. Utilizing Relaxation Techniques:

   - Incorporating relaxation techniques, such as progressive muscle relaxation or guided imagery, contributes to emotional resilience. These techniques not only alleviate physical tension but also promote a sense of calm and balance, enhancing the ability to cope with the emotional impact of migraines.

12. Celebrating Small Wins:

- Acknowledging and celebrating small victories, even amidst the challenges of migraines, nurtures resilience. Recognizing achievements, no matter how modest, reinforces a positive mindset and encourages a proactive approach to managing migraines.

13. Building Emotional Intelligence:

- Developing emotional intelligence involves recognizing, understanding, and managing one's own emotions. Building emotional intelligence enhances resilience by promoting effective coping strategies, fostering empathy for oneself, and navigating interpersonal relationships with greater ease.

14. Gratitude Practices:

- Cultivating gratitude through regular practices, such as keeping a gratitude journal, contributes to resilience. Focusing on positive aspects of life, even in the presence of migraines, fosters a mindset of appreciation and resilience in the face of adversity.

15. Engaging in Self-Care:

- Prioritizing self-care is a cornerstone of resilience. Engaging in activities that promote physical, mental, and emotional well-being, such as taking breaks, practicing self-compassion, and setting boundaries, contributes to an overall resilient approach to living with migraines.

In conclusion, building resilience in the face of migraines is a dynamic and ongoing process that involves a combination of psychological, emotional, and lifestyle strategies. By incorporating these strategies into their lives, individuals can enhance their capacity to adapt, endure, and thrive despite the challenges presented by chronic headache

CHAPTER 9

SUPPORT SYSTEM

A support system is a vital network of relationships, whether comprised of friends, family, colleagues, or community, that provides emotional, practical, and often indispensable assistance during challenging times. This interconnected web of support serves as a cornerstone for individual well-being, offering empathy, encouragement, and understanding. In the face of life's complexities, having a robust support system becomes an invaluable resource, providing a sense of belonging, shared experiences, and a collaborative foundation for navigating difficulties. This network not only bolsters individuals during times of hardship but also fosters a sense of community and connection that contributes to emotional resilience and personal growth.

THE ROLE OF FAMILY AND FRIENDS

Family and friends play a pivotal role in shaping our lives, offering unwavering support, love, and companionship that extend beyond the ordinary rhythms of daily existence. In times of both joy and challenge, the significance of this support network becomes particularly evident. Within the context of health struggles, such as dealing with migraines, the role of family and friends takes on added importance.

First and foremost, family provides a foundational pillar of support. The intimate bonds forged through shared experiences and familial connections create a unique reservoir of understanding. For someone navigating the complexities of migraines, having family members who empathize with the physical and emotional toll of chronic headaches is invaluable. The familial support system often involves practical assistance, such as helping with household tasks during migraine episodes, but extends far beyond, encompassing emotional encouragement and an unwavering commitment to the individual's well-being.

Friends, on the other hand, constitute a chosen family, a community of companions who contribute to the mosaic of life. In the realm of health challenges, friends serve as empathetic listeners, offering understanding and companionship during moments of vulnerability. Their role extends beyond the immediate challenges of migraines, contributing to the creation of a positive and nurturing environment that promotes overall well-being.

The significance of family and friends lies not only in their capacity to provide assistance but also in their ability to foster resilience. The emotional support offered by loved ones becomes a beacon of strength, enabling individuals to face the uncertainties associated with health conditions with greater courage and determination. Moreover, the shared moments of joy, laughter, and mutual support create bonds that transcend the specific challenges of migraines, contributing to a sense of belonging and community.

In essence, the role of family and friends in the context of health challenges is multifaceted. They serve as pillars of strength, sources of practical assistance, and catalysts for emotional resilience. Together, they form an integral part of an individual's journey, shaping the narrative of living with migraines and providing a foundation upon which one can navigate the complexities of life with a chronic health condition.

CONNECTING WITH MIGRAINE COMMUNITY

Connecting with the migraine community is a powerful and transformative journey that offers individuals living with migraines a sense of solidarity, understanding, and shared experiences. This community, often found online and in various support groups, serves as a valuable resource for information, emotional support, and a platform for exchanging coping strategies. This exploration delves into the significance of connecting with the migraine community and the myriad ways in which this shared experience fosters a sense of belonging and empowerment.

1. Shared Understanding:
   - One of the primary benefits of connecting with the migraine community is the shared understanding that comes from individuals who are navigating similar challenges. Within this community, experiences that might be difficult to convey to those without migraines are met with empathy and understanding, creating a space where individuals feel seen and heard.

2. Information and Resources:

   - The migraine community serves as a rich source of information and resources. From the latest research on migraine treatments to practical tips for managing symptoms, the collective knowledge within the community empowers individuals with valuable insights. Online forums, social media groups, and dedicated websites provide platforms for sharing experiences and staying informed about developments in migraine research and treatment.

3. Emotional Support:

   - Living with migraines can be emotionally taxing, and the migraine community offers a virtual embrace where individuals can share their triumphs, frustrations, and vulnerabilities. This emotional support is crucial for mental well-being, providing a safe space to express feelings, seek advice, and receive encouragement from those who understand the unique challenges associated with migraines.

4. Coping Strategies:

   - The community becomes a treasure trove of coping strategies. Individuals share their personal approaches to managing migraines, ranging from relaxation techniques to lifestyle adjustments. This exchange of practical advice allows community members to discover strategies that resonate with their unique experiences, enhancing their ability to cope with the impact of migraines.

5. Empowerment through Advocacy:

   - Connecting with the migraine community often sparks a sense of empowerment through advocacy. Many individuals find their voice and a platform for raising awareness about migraines, challenging misconceptions, and advocating for improved understanding and support. Collective advocacy efforts contribute to reducing stigma and promoting a more inclusive environment for those living with migraines.

6. Building a Support Network:

   - The migraine community becomes a virtual support network. Individuals forge connections that extend beyond the digital realm, creating bonds that provide reassurance and understanding. These connections offer a lifeline during challenging times, fostering a sense of community that transcends the geographical distances that may separate members.

7. Education and Awareness:
   - Participating in the migraine community contributes to ongoing education and awareness. Individuals become more informed about the diverse nature of migraines, different treatment approaches, and the impact of lifestyle factors. This knowledge not only benefits individuals personally but also equips them to educate others and contribute to dispelling myths surrounding migraines.

8. Reducing Isolation:
   - Migraines can be isolating, and the community serves as a powerful antidote to this isolation. By connecting with others who share similar experiences, individuals realize that they are not alone in their journey. This realization is profoundly liberating and diminishes the sense of isolation that migraines can often induce.

9. Validation of Experiences:
   - Within the migraine community, individuals find validation for their experiences. The challenges and triumphs shared by others resonate deeply, affirming the legitimacy of each person's journey with migraines. This validation contributes to a sense of self-acceptance and acknowledgment within the community.

10. Opportunities for Collaboration:
   - Connecting with the migraine community opens doors for collaboration. Whether it's participating in research initiatives, contributing personal stories to awareness campaigns, or sharing advocacy efforts, community members find opportunities to collaborate and make a collective impact in the larger landscape of migraine awareness and support.

In conclusion, connecting with the migraine community is a transformative experience that transcends the digital realm. It provides individuals with a sense of belonging, a wealth of information and resources, emotional support, and a platform for advocacy. By forging connections within this community, individuals living with migraines enhance their resilience, find empowerment, and contribute to a collective effort to improve understanding and support for everyone impacted by migraines.

CONCLUSION

In concluding the insightful journey through "Managing and Understanding Migraine: A Clear Path to Navigating and Controlling Migraine," the pages have unfolded as a roadmap for individuals seeking not just relief but a comprehensive understanding of migraines. This book has aspired to be a guiding light, offering clarity, practical solutions, and a sense of empowerment for those navigating the intricate landscape of migraines.

From the foundational understanding of migraine anatomy to the nuanced exploration of triggers, types, and treatments, the book has aimed to equip readers with the knowledge necessary to demystify this complex condition. The emphasis on setting realistic goals, tracking migraine patterns, and creating personalized management plans underscores the individualized nature of the migraine journey.

Throughout these chapters, the importance of a holistic approach has been a recurring theme. Beyond pharmaceutical interventions, lifestyle adjustments, emotional well-being, and connecting with the migraine community have emerged as essential pillars in the pursuit of headache harmony. By offering tools for recognizing triggers, understanding symptoms, and navigating the often unpredictable course of migraines, this book seeks to empower individuals to take charge of their well-being.

In conclusion, the narrative of "Managing and Understanding Migraine" is one of empowerment and resilience. It recognizes the challenges inherent in living with migraines but contends that with knowledge, support, and personalized strategies, individuals can forge a path towards control and stability. May this book serve not just as a reference but as a companion on the journey towards managing migraines, providing insights, reassurance, and practical guidance for those seeking clarity and control over this often debilitating condition. May it be a beacon of hope, offering a clear path to navigate and ultimately triumph over the challenges of living with migraines.

www.ingramcontent.com/pod-product-compliance
Lightning Source LLC
Chambersburg PA
CBHW070947290526
45795CB00005B/1670